Ben Andrews' BETTER PLACES

Nicky and Candy's Street

Illustrated by Charlotte Jenkins

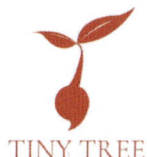

TINY TREE

In memory of my mum,
'Nicky' Nicola Andrews

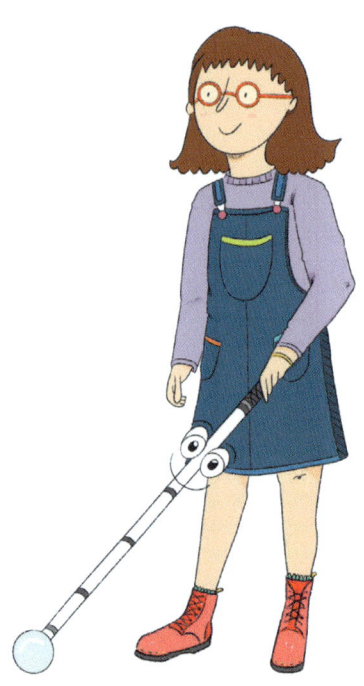

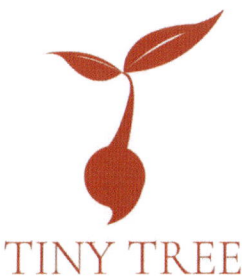

TINY TREE

First Published in 2023
Tiny Tree (an imprint of Andrews UK Limited)

West Wing Studios, Unit 166, The Mall, Luton, Beds, LU1 2TL

www.tinytreebooks.com

ISBN: 978-1-837913-83-1

Text copyright © 2023 Ben Andrews
The moral rights of the author(s) have been asserted.

Apart from any fair dealing for the purpose of research, or private study, or criticism or review as permitted under the Copyright, Designs and Patents Act, 1988, this publication may only be reproduced, stored or transmitted in any form, or by any means, with the prior permission of the publisher, or in the case of reprographic reproduction, in accordance with the terms of licenses issued by the Copyright Licensing Agency. Enquiries concerning reproduction outside those terms should be sent to the publisher.

Illustrations copyright © 2023 Charlotte Jenkins

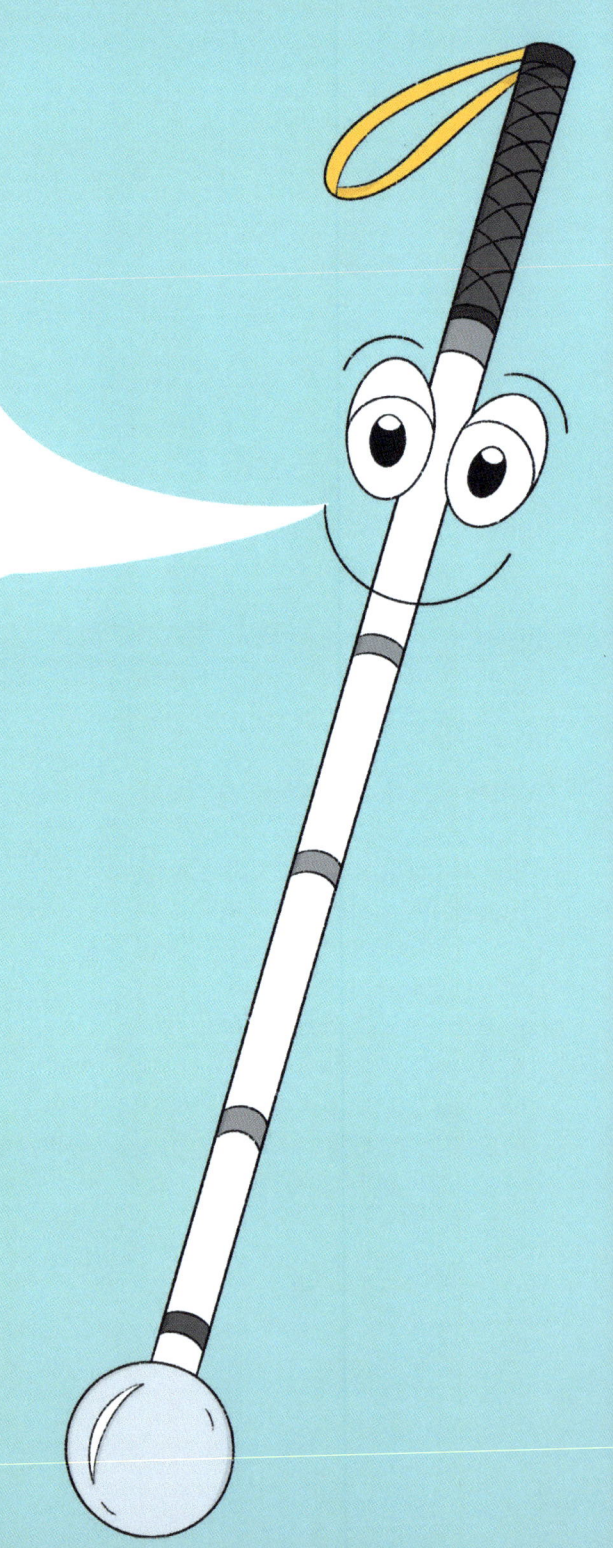

"Hey, I'm Candy.
Great to meet you.
I'm a tall, thin white cane.
Nicky uses me to get around.

Nicky swings me
from left to right
and I let Nicky know
if there's something
in front of her.
We're a great team.

But places aren't
always that great.
They can make
getting around hard.

I know, why don't we
work together to make…"

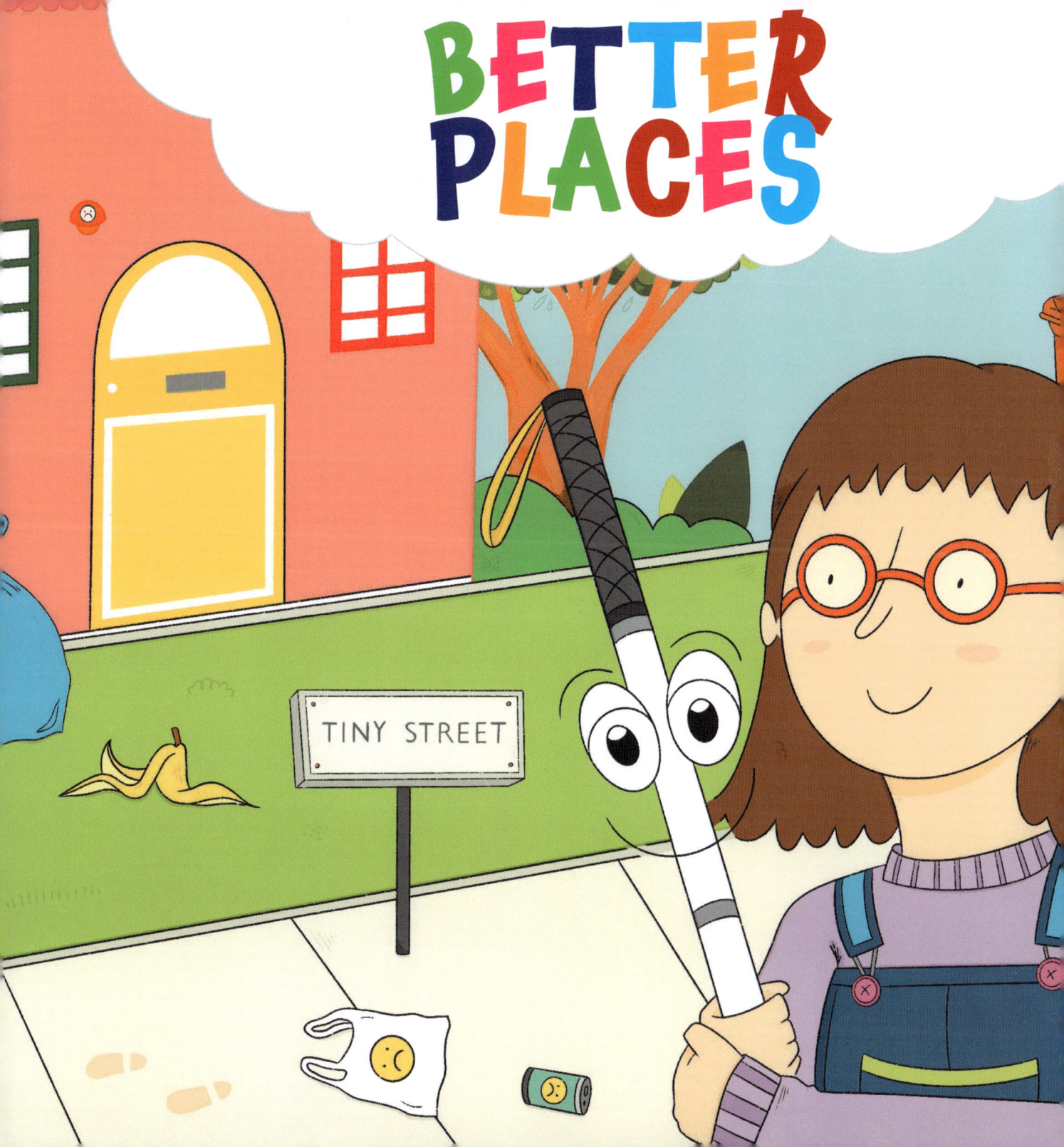

Nicky was going to see their friend, Kim.

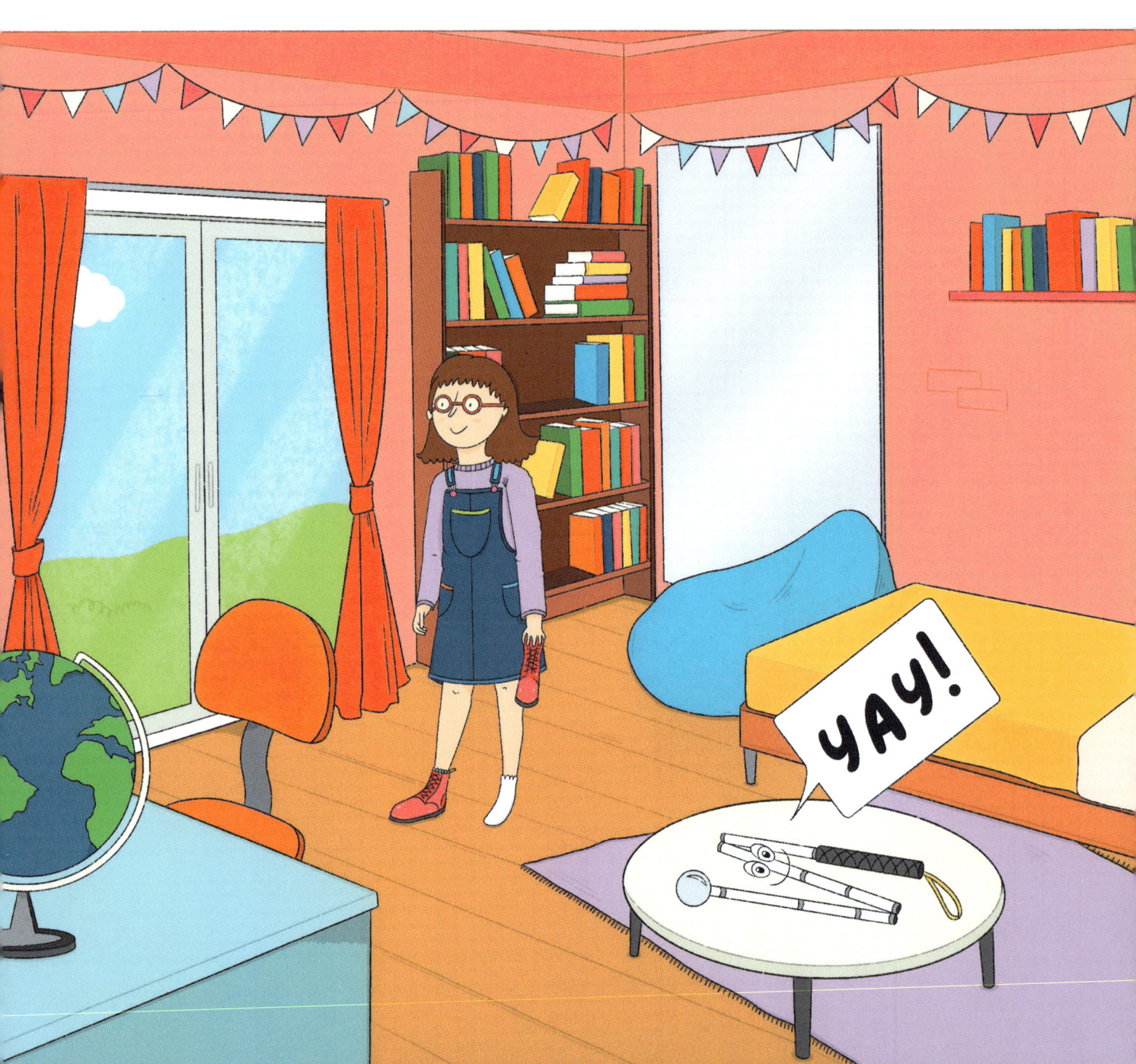

But Kim lived very far away.
All the way at the other end of the street, in fact.

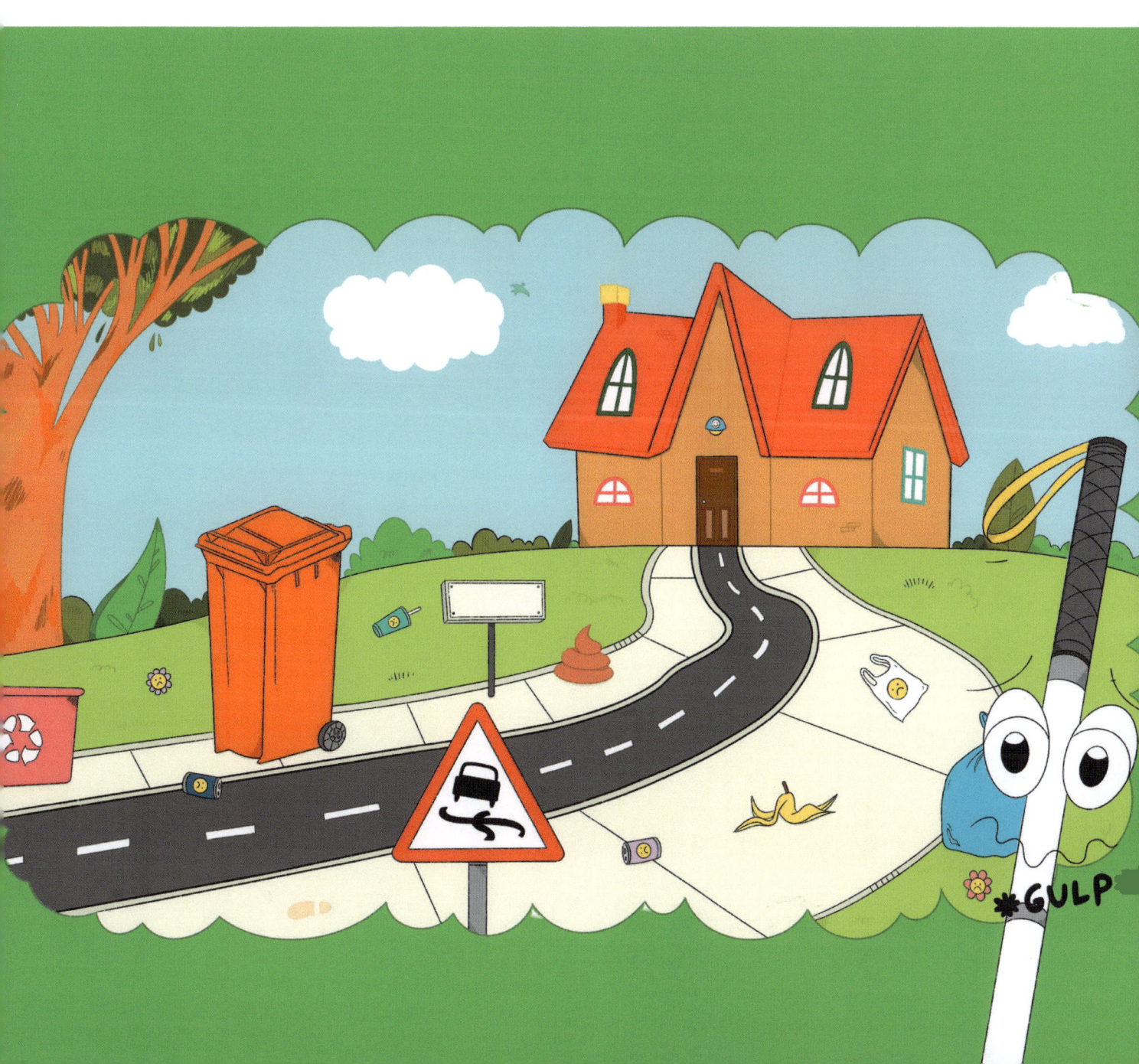

Getting down the street wasn't easy.
As soon as Nicky left the house, Candy was...

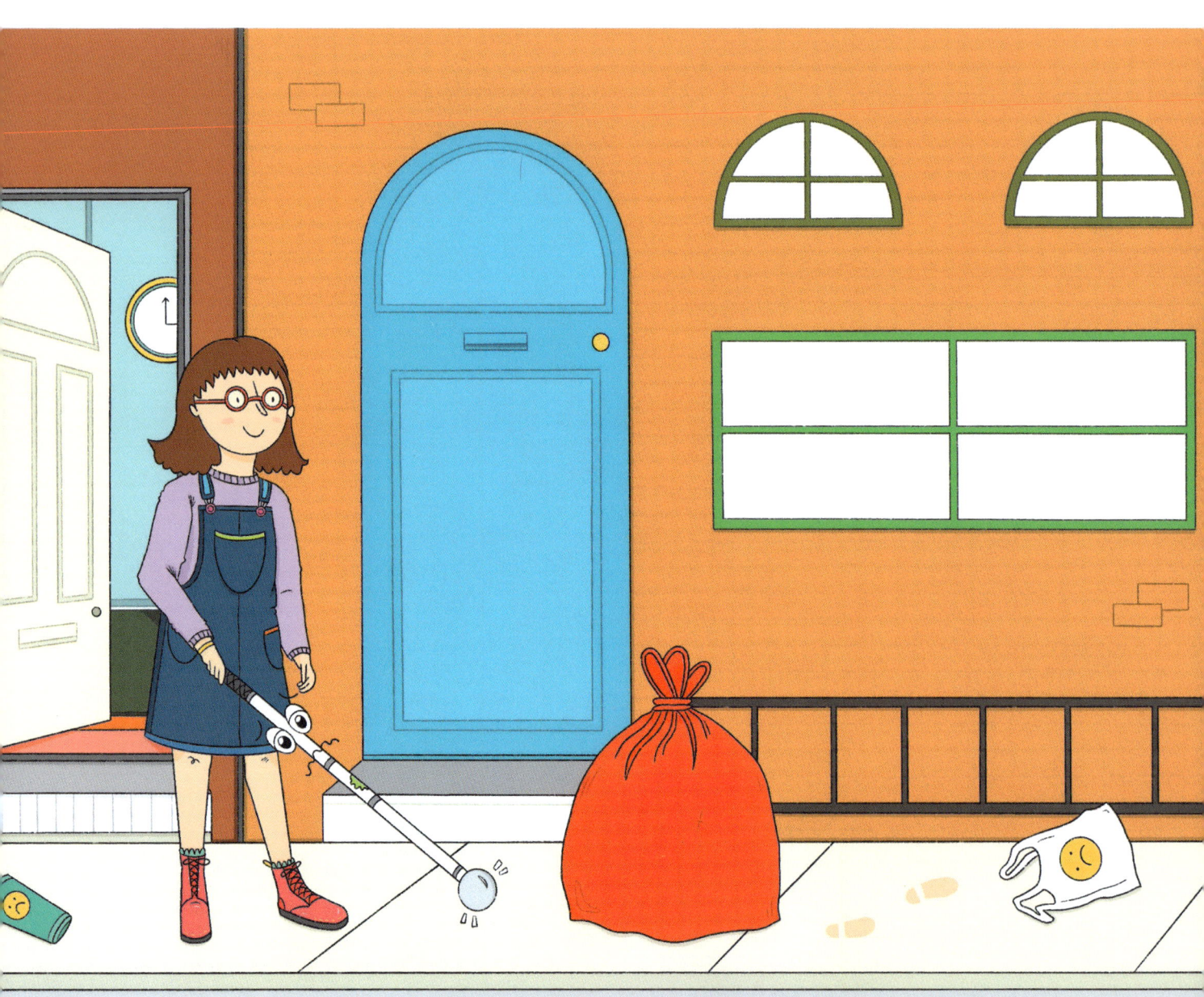

swished and swooshed into stinky rubbish bins and bags,

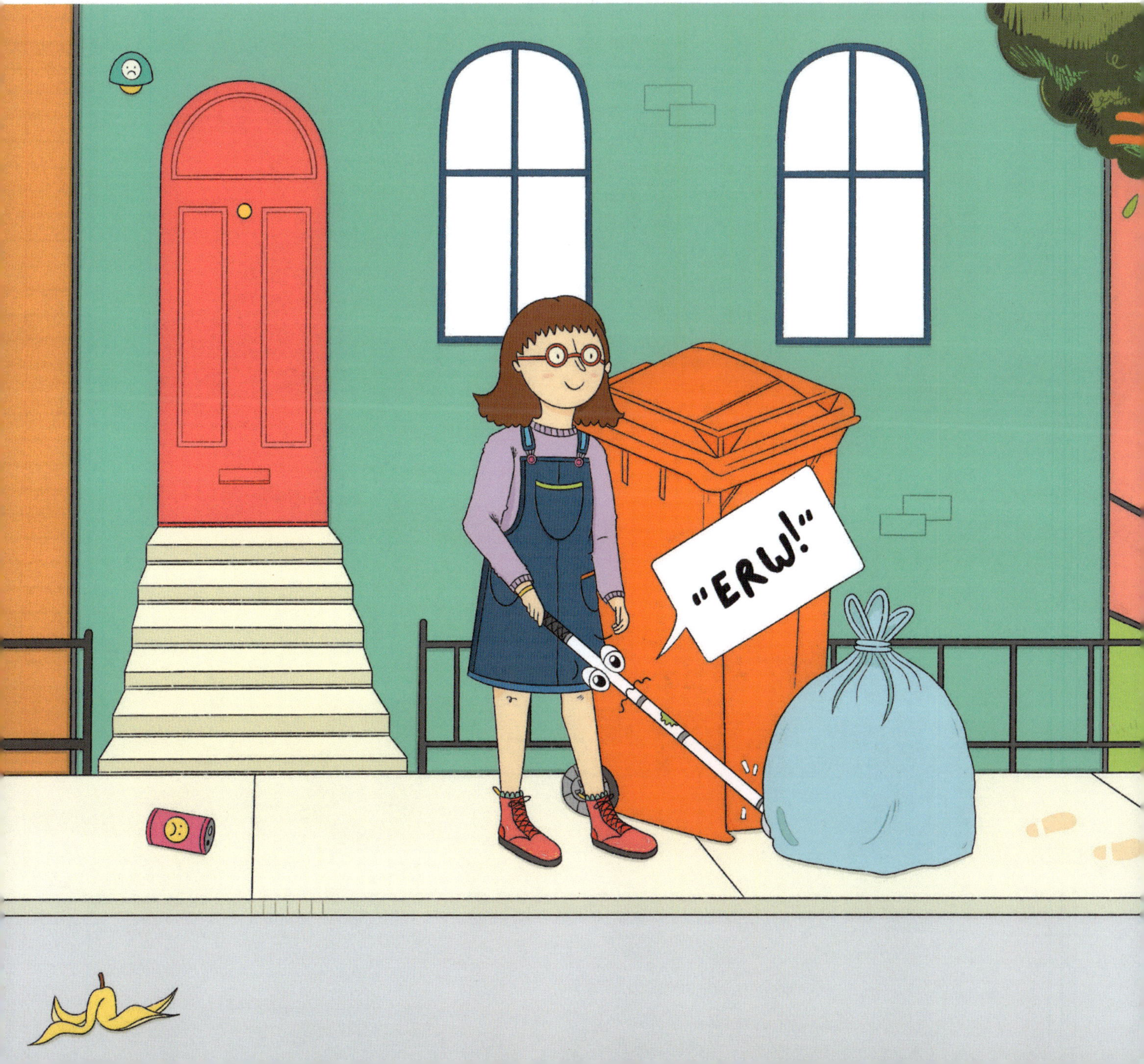

banged and bumped into oddly placed signs, posts, and trees,

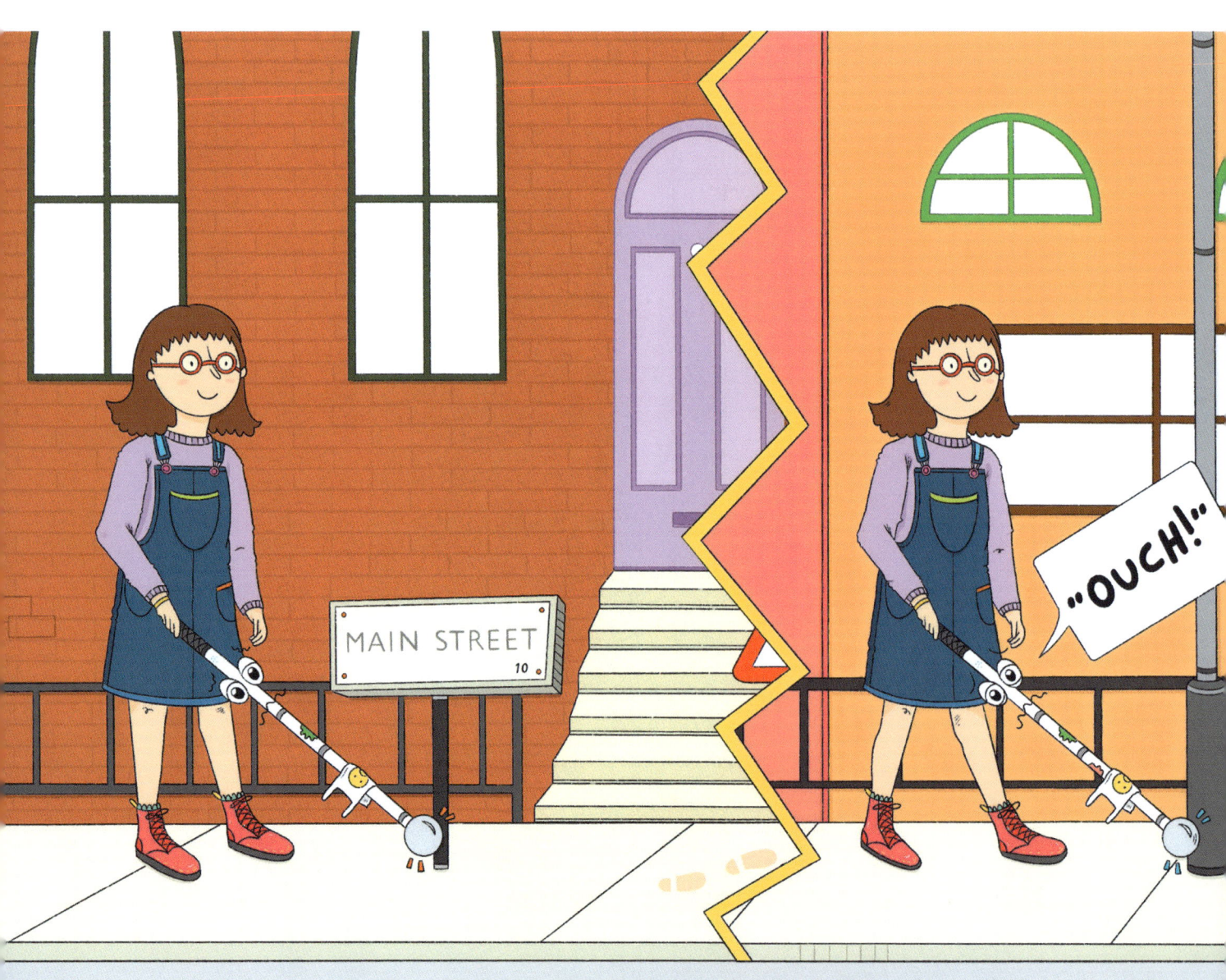

and worst of all, just as they reached Kim's garden...

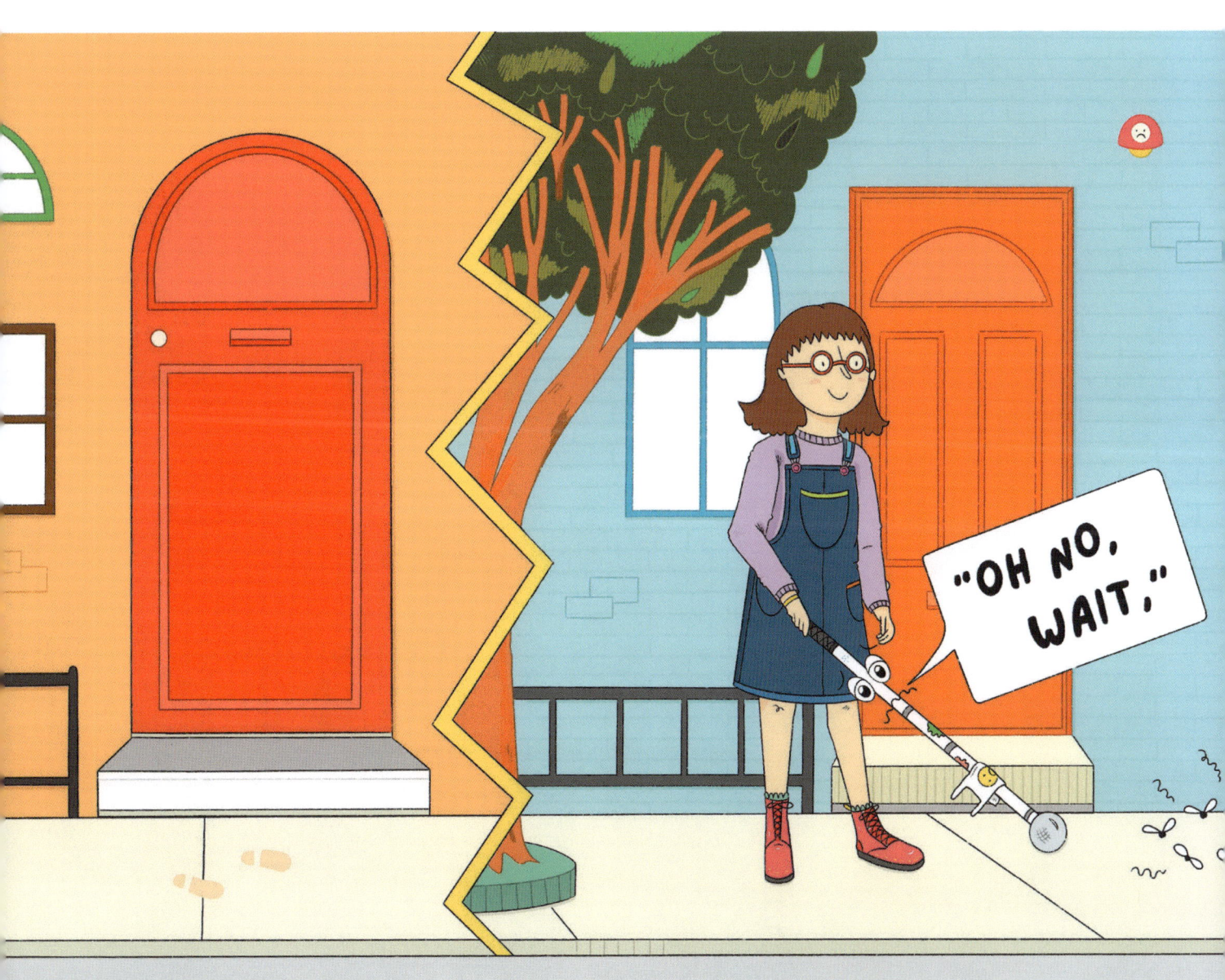

Candy was swung into a big pile of smelly dog poop.

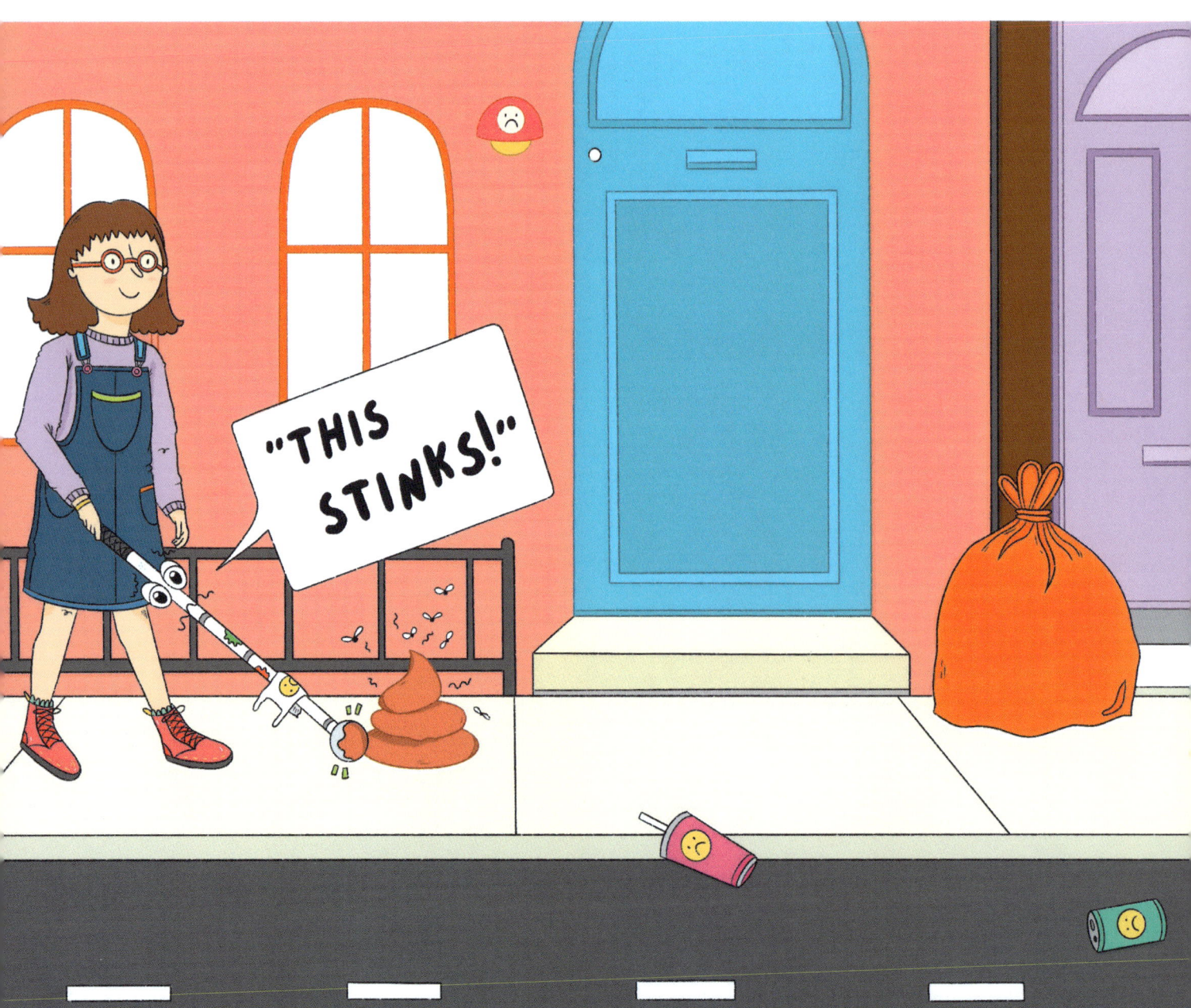

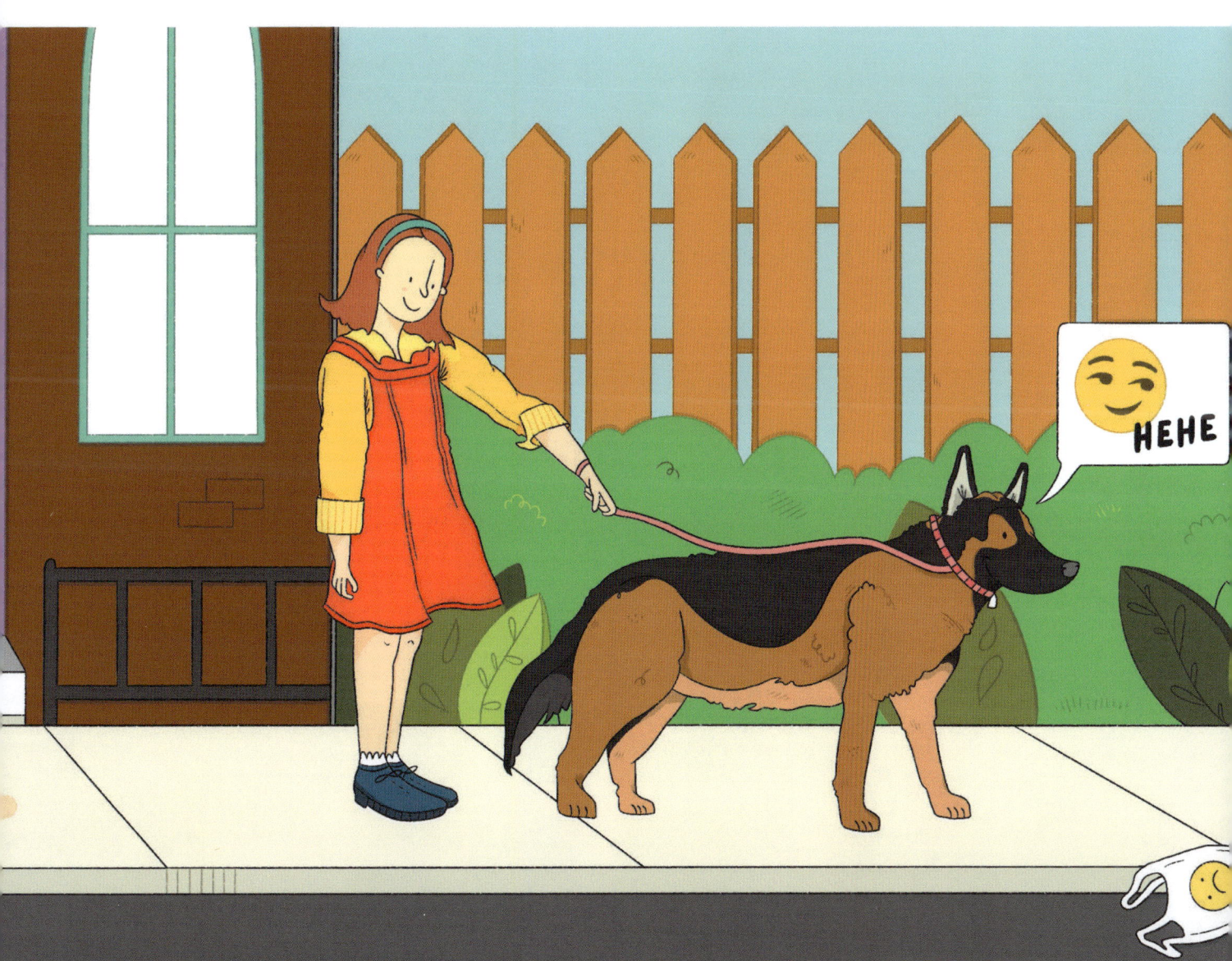

Finally, they made it to Kim's house, where they played all sorts of fun games.

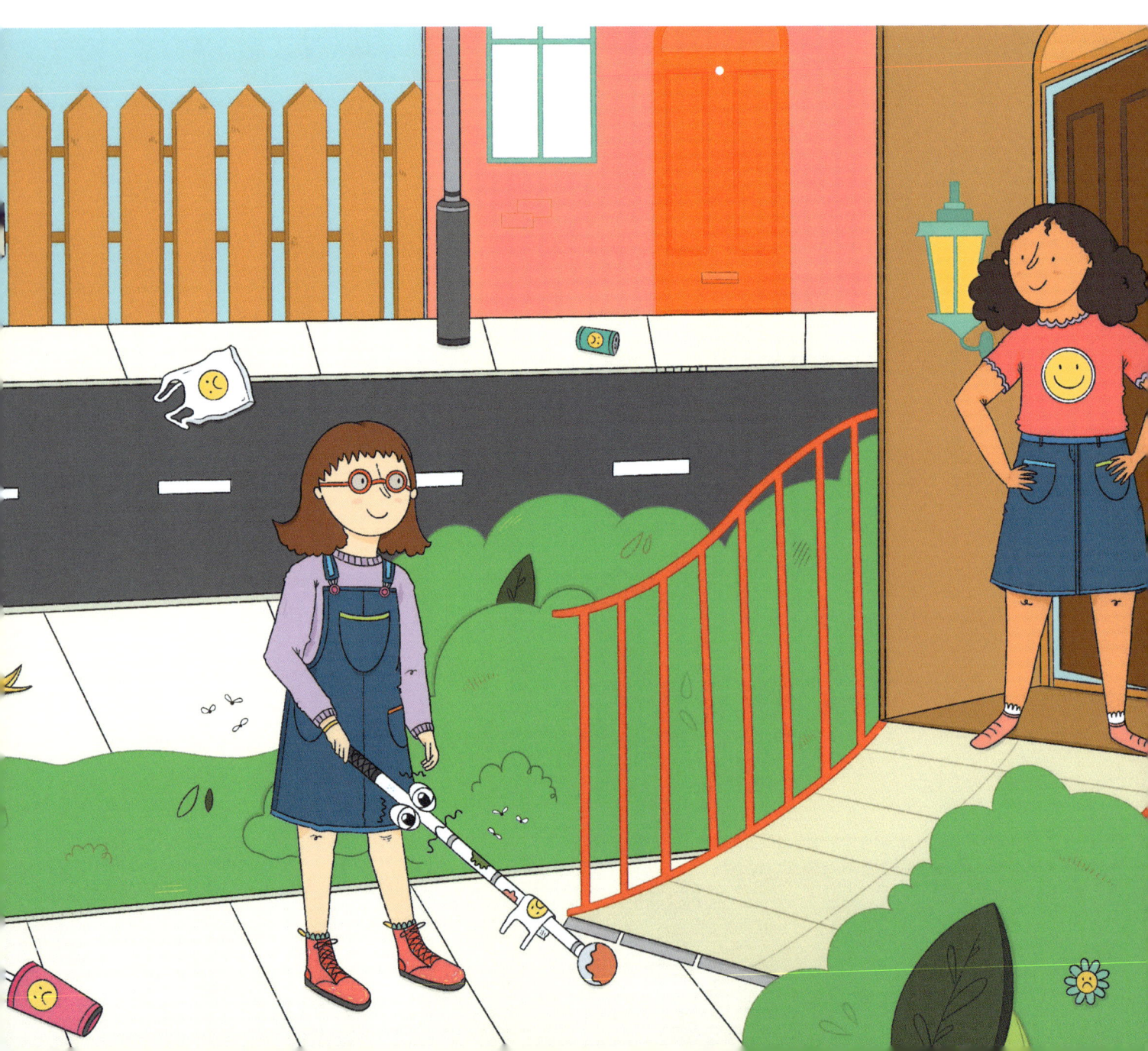

From limbo in the loft,

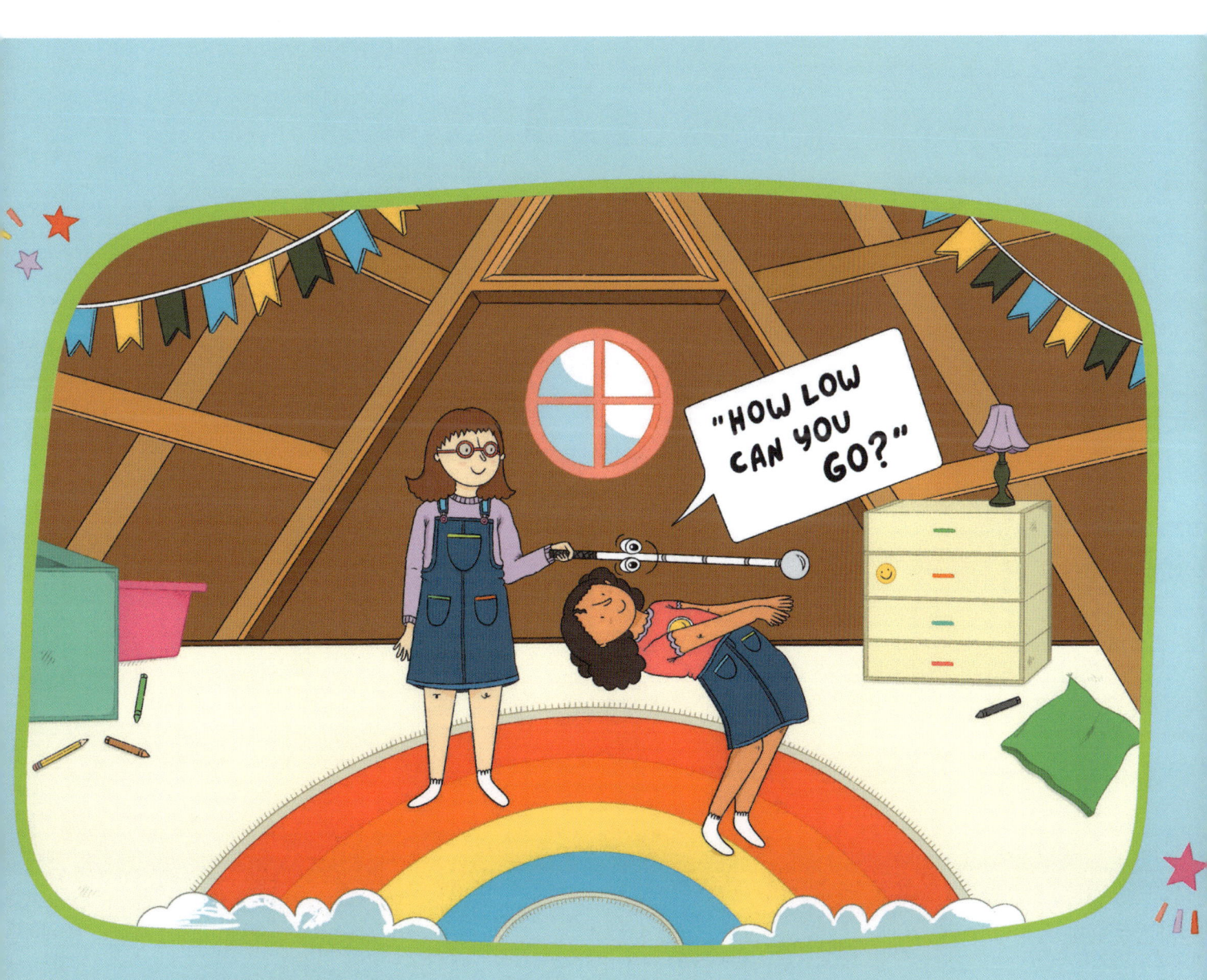

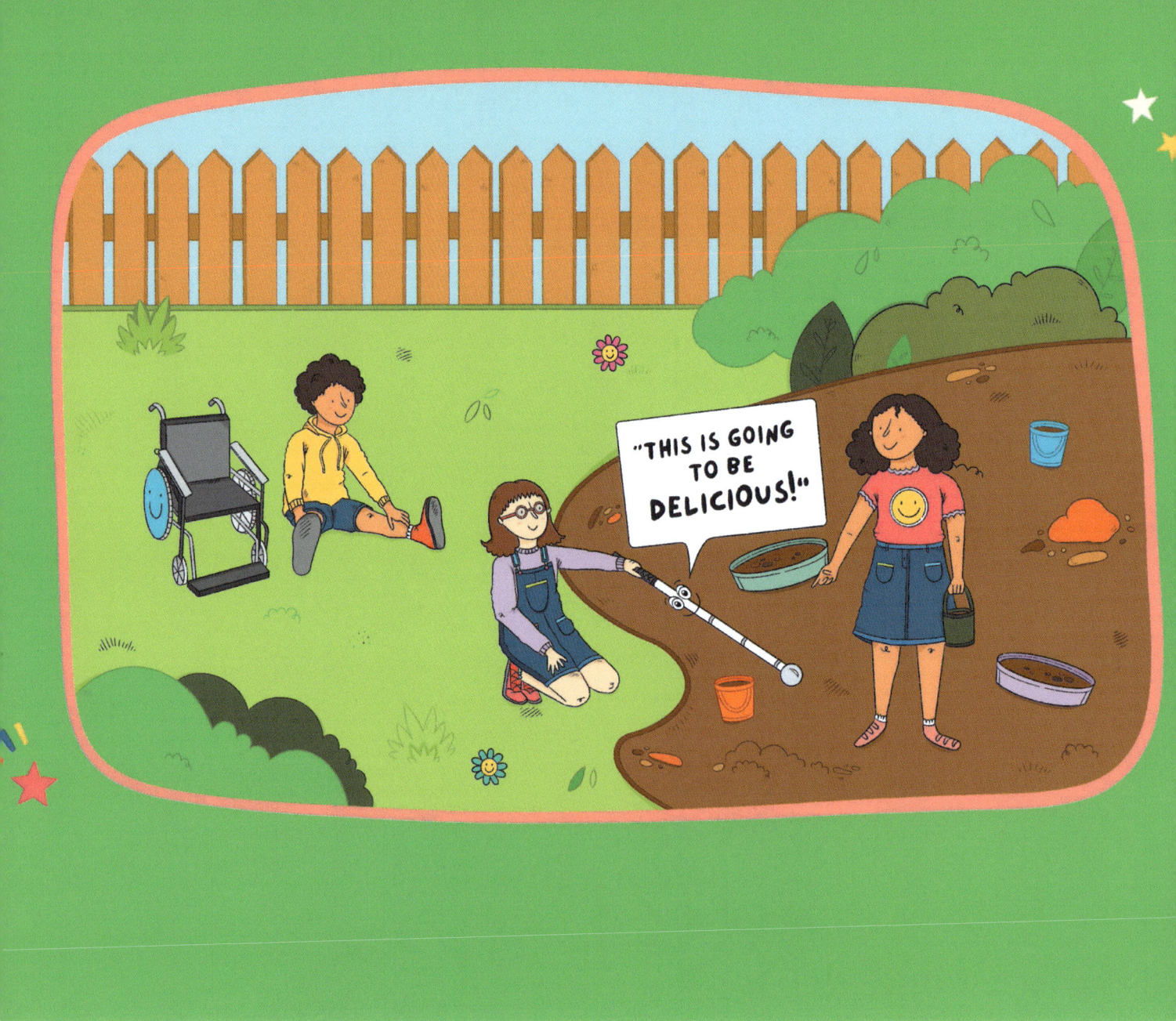

to making mud pies on the patio,

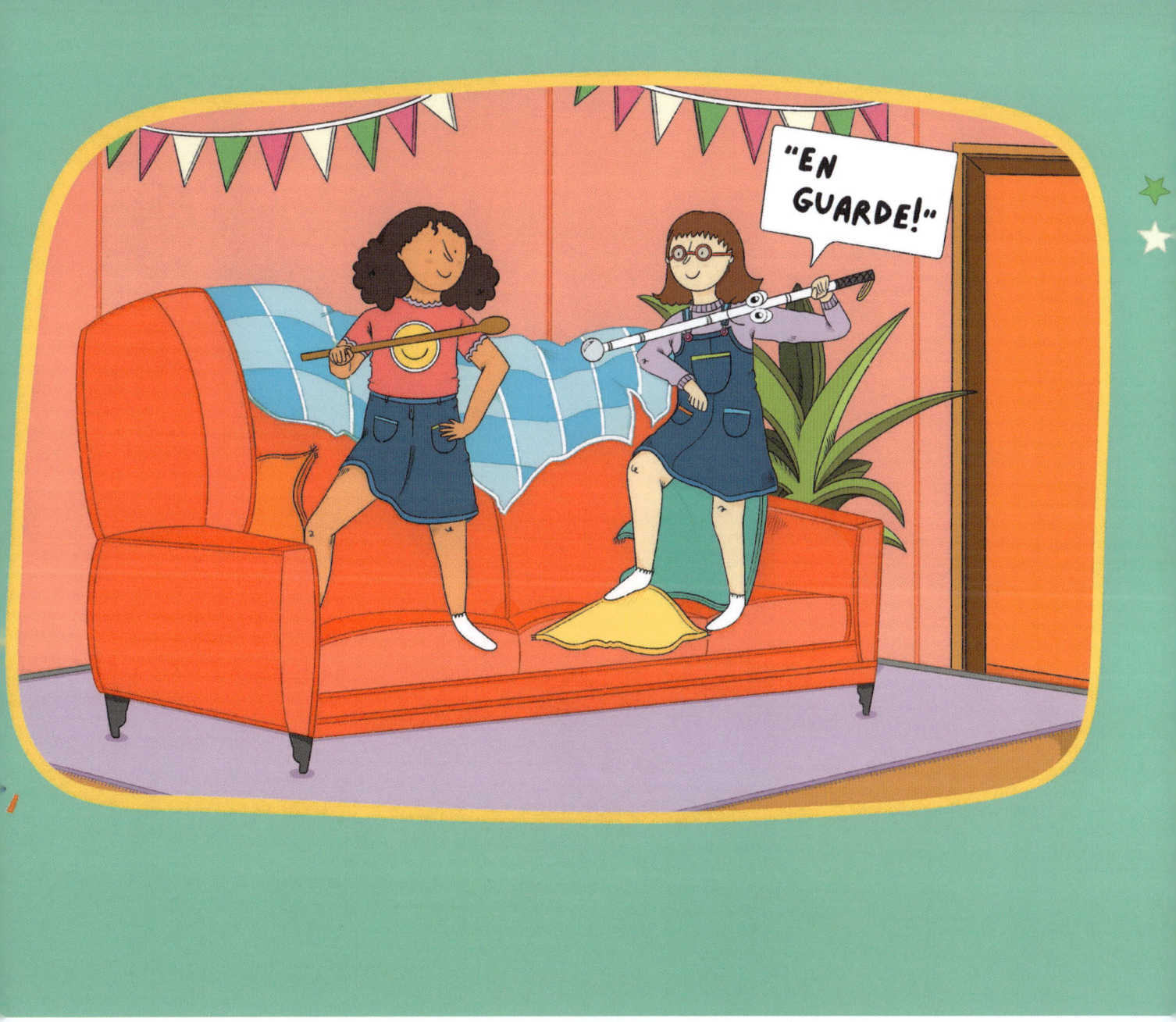

and sword fights on the sofa.

But before they knew it, it was time to go home.

Candy didn't want to go back outside.

It was dirty, painful, and smelly.

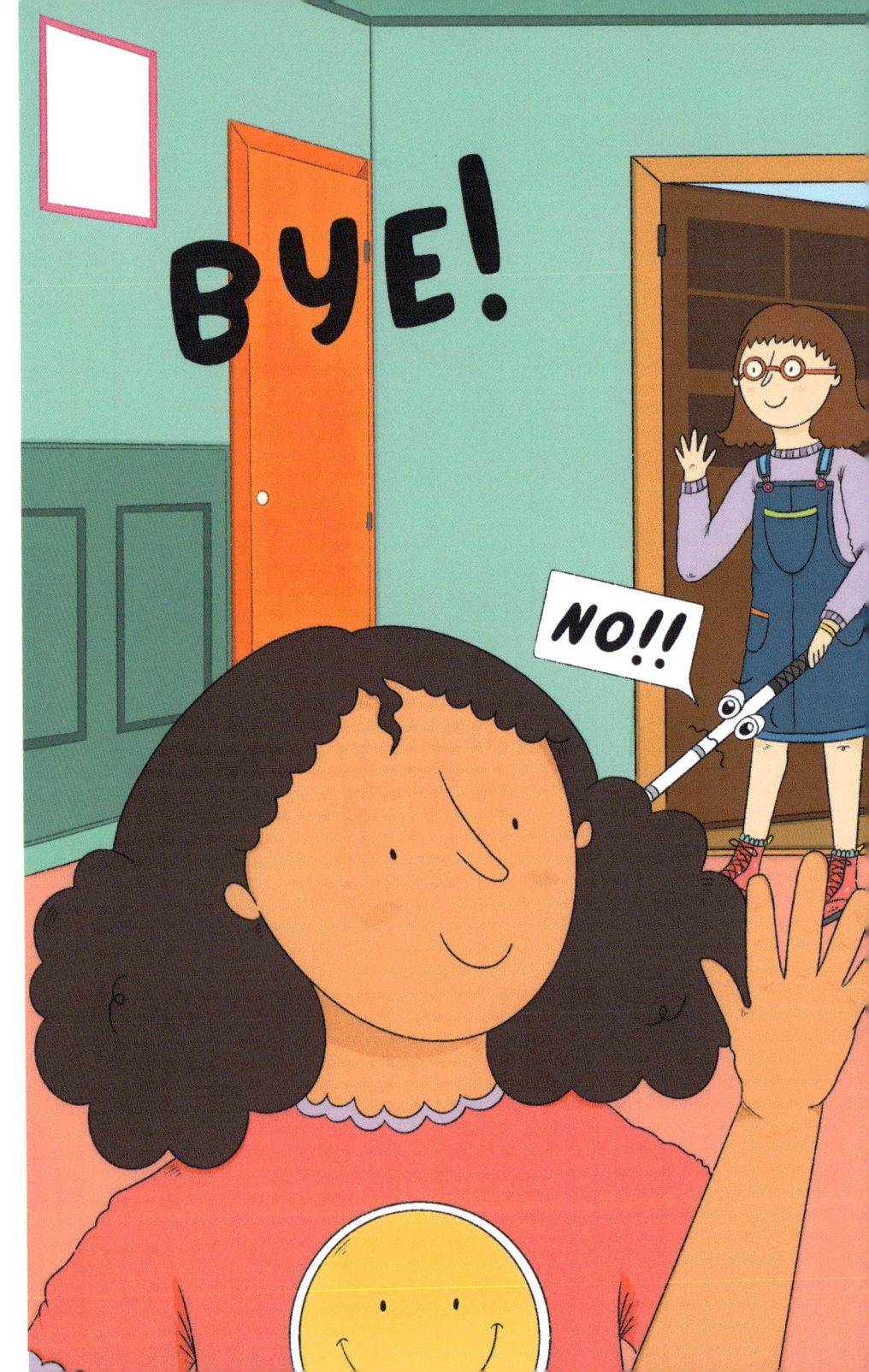

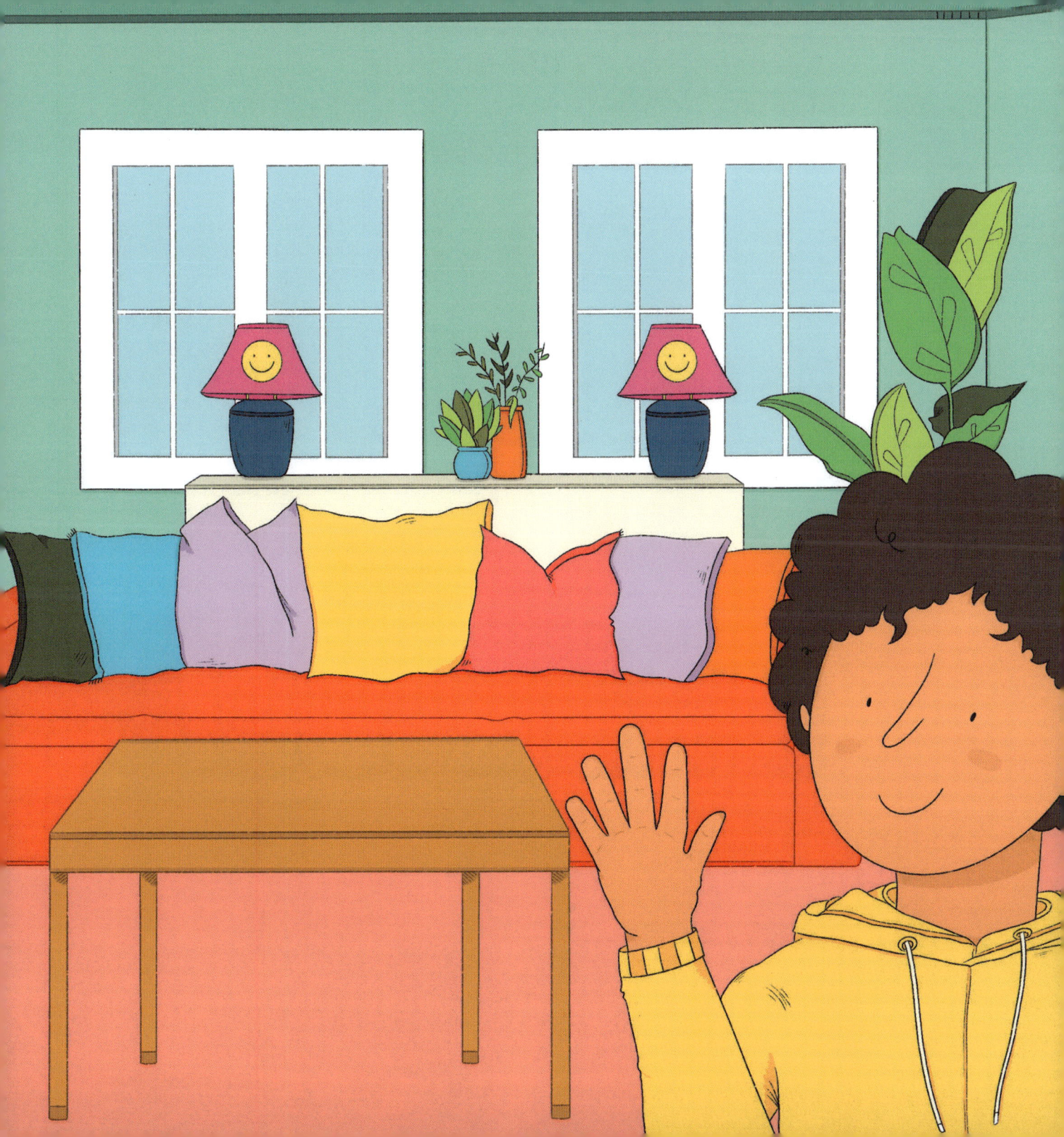

Now's our chance.
Let's work together to make the street a
BETTER PLACE.

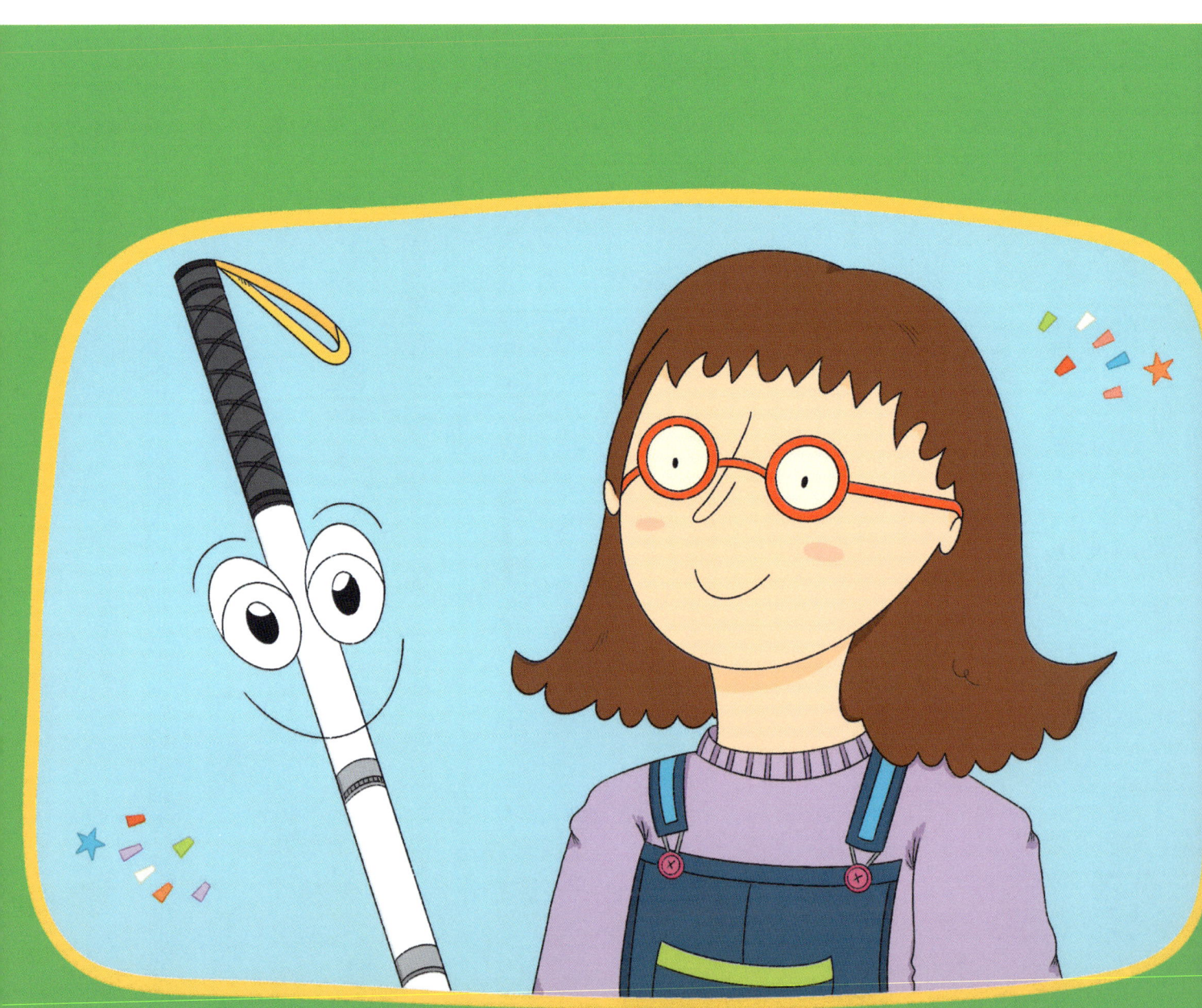

First, let's pick up the poop and put it in the bin.

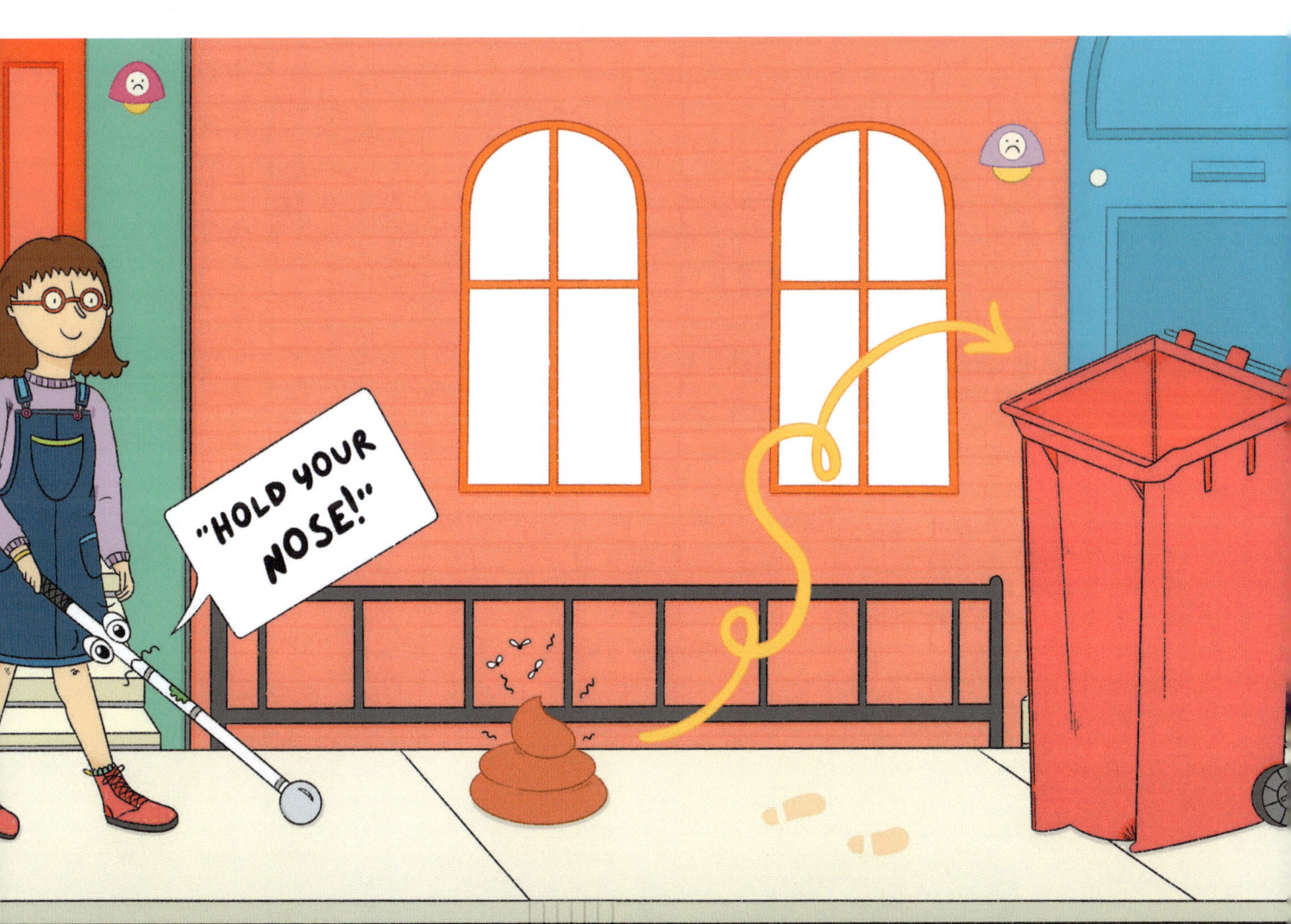

Quick! Let's turn the page to see if it's worked.

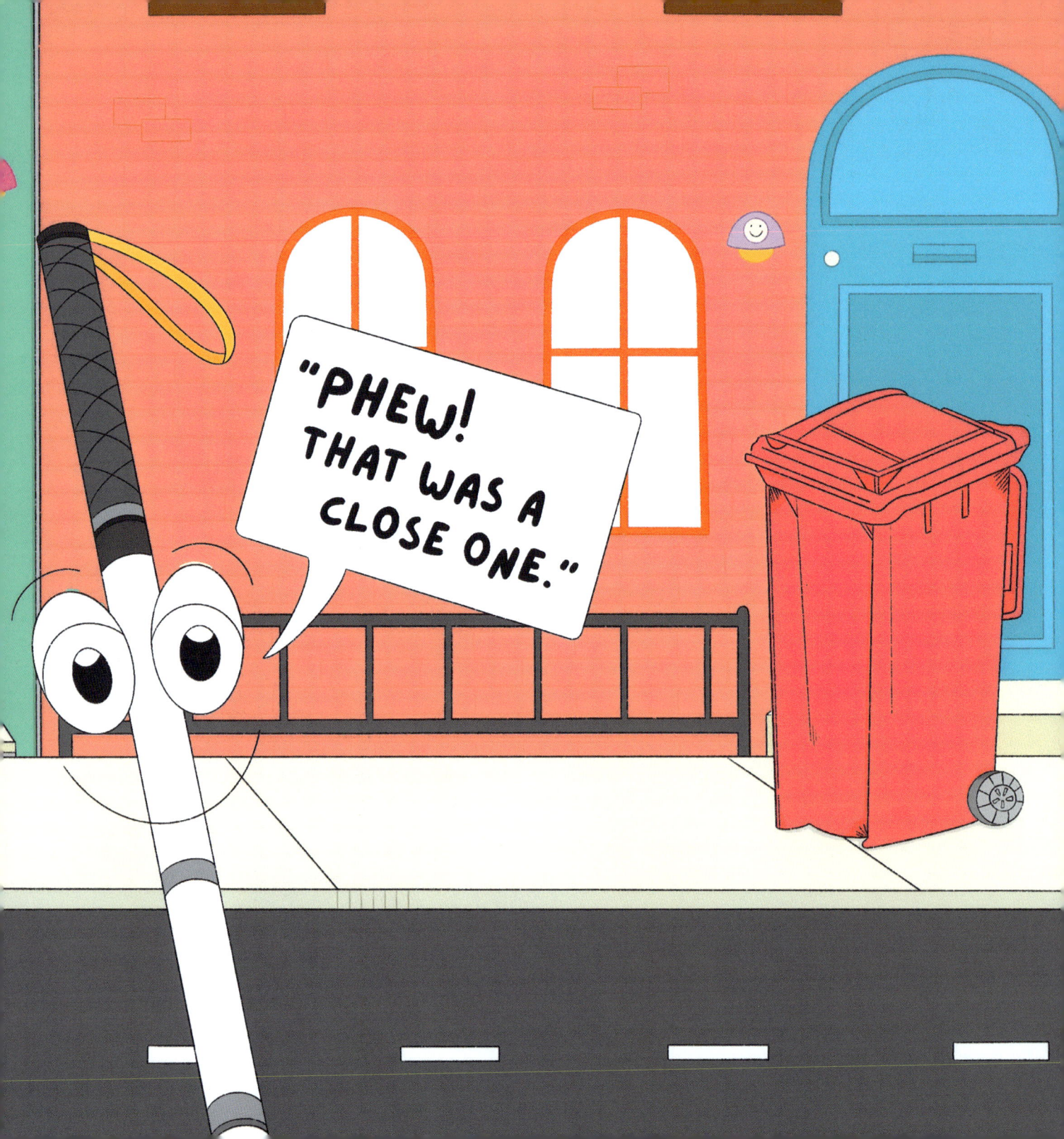

Now let's flick all of those oddly placed things out of the way.

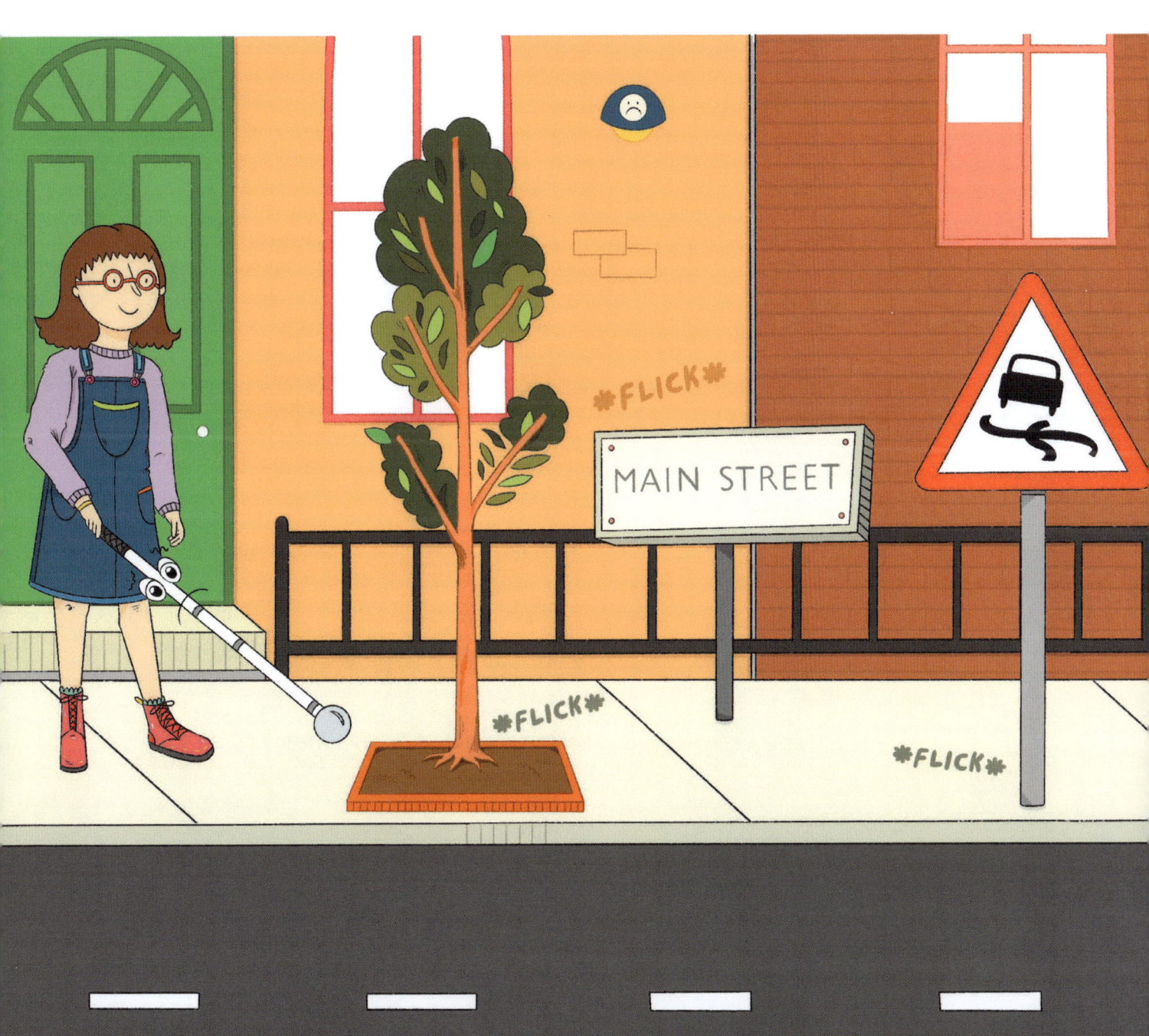

Ah. Everything in the right place.

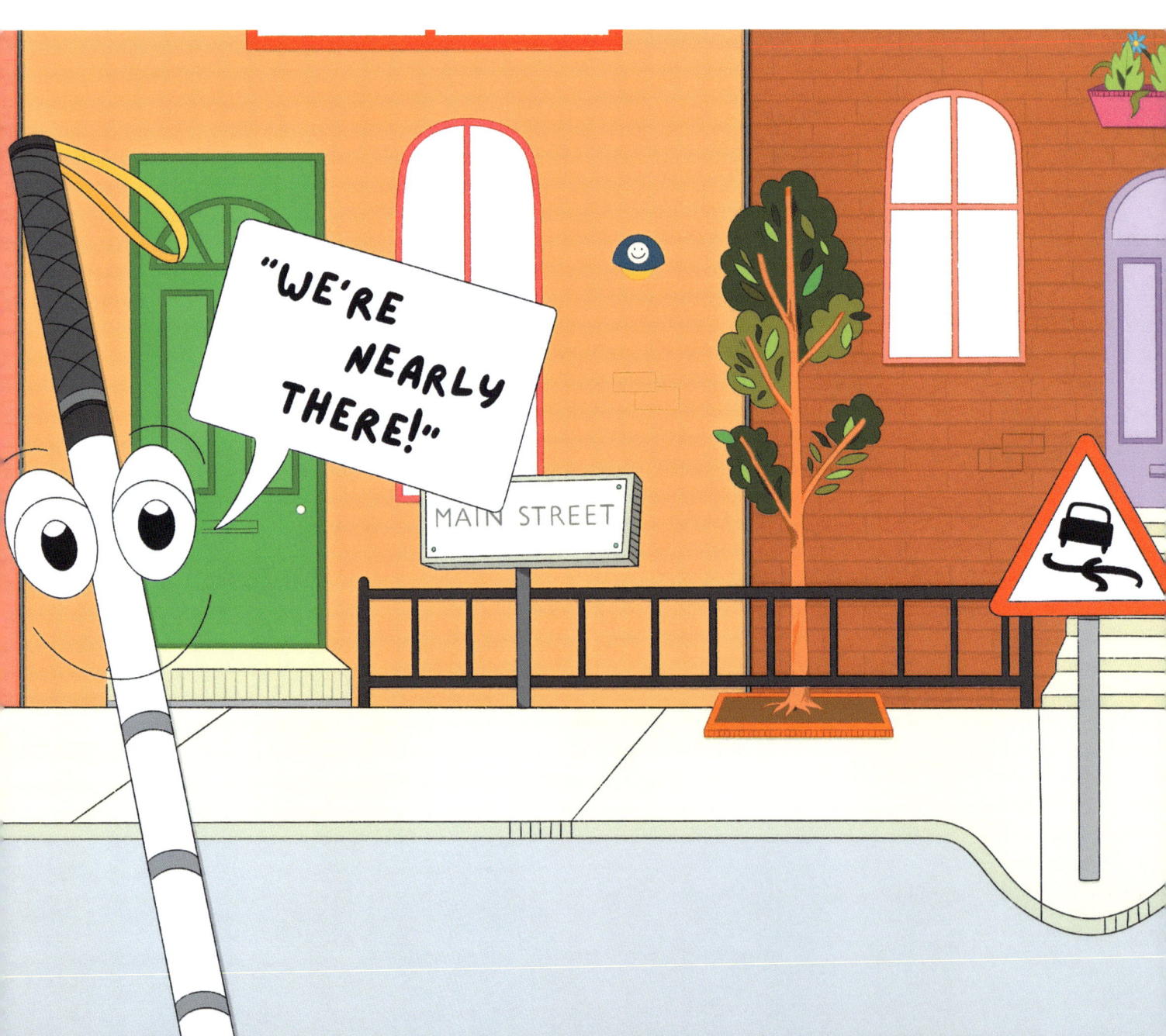

Let's pull all those rubbish bins and bags somewhere safe.

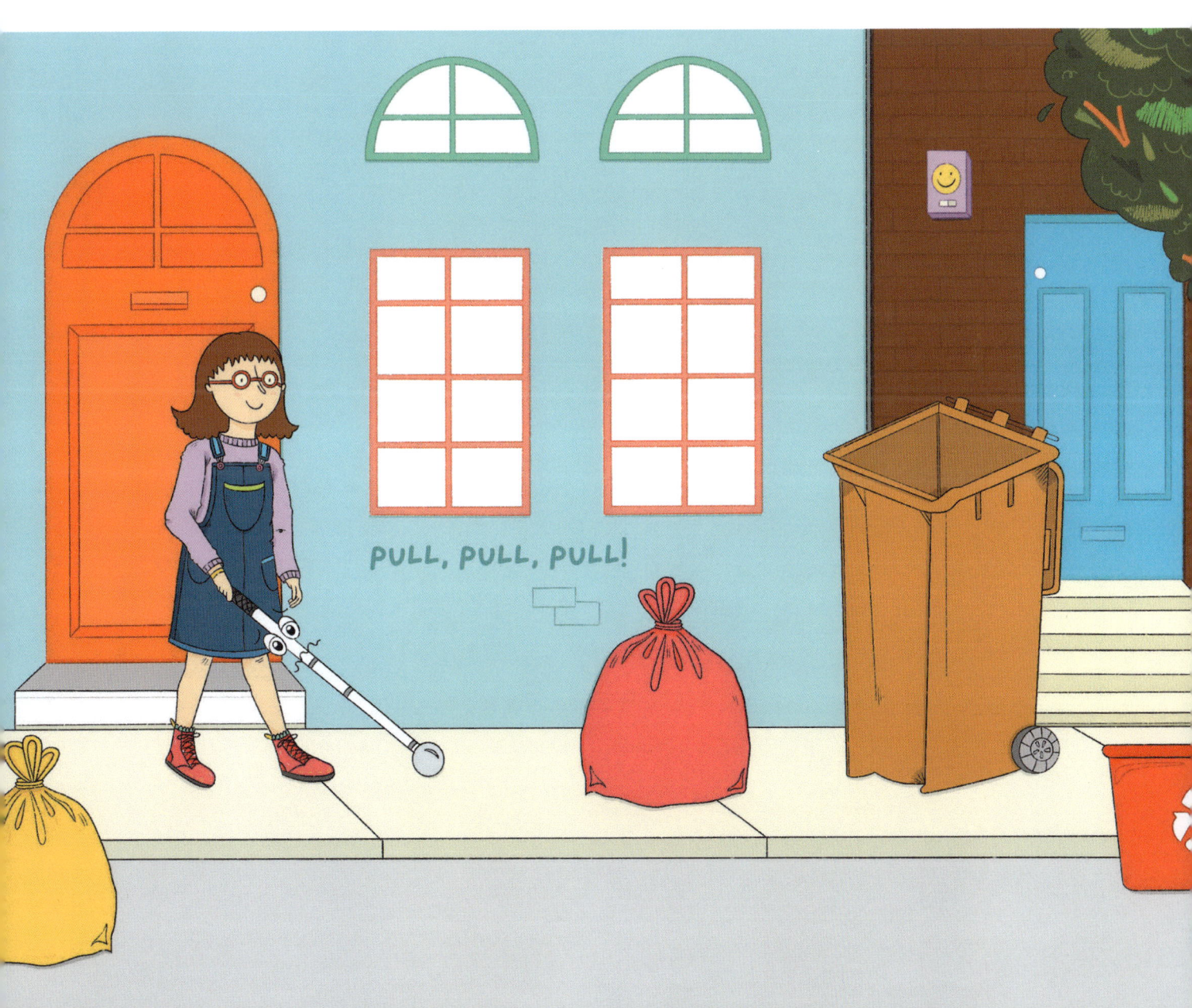

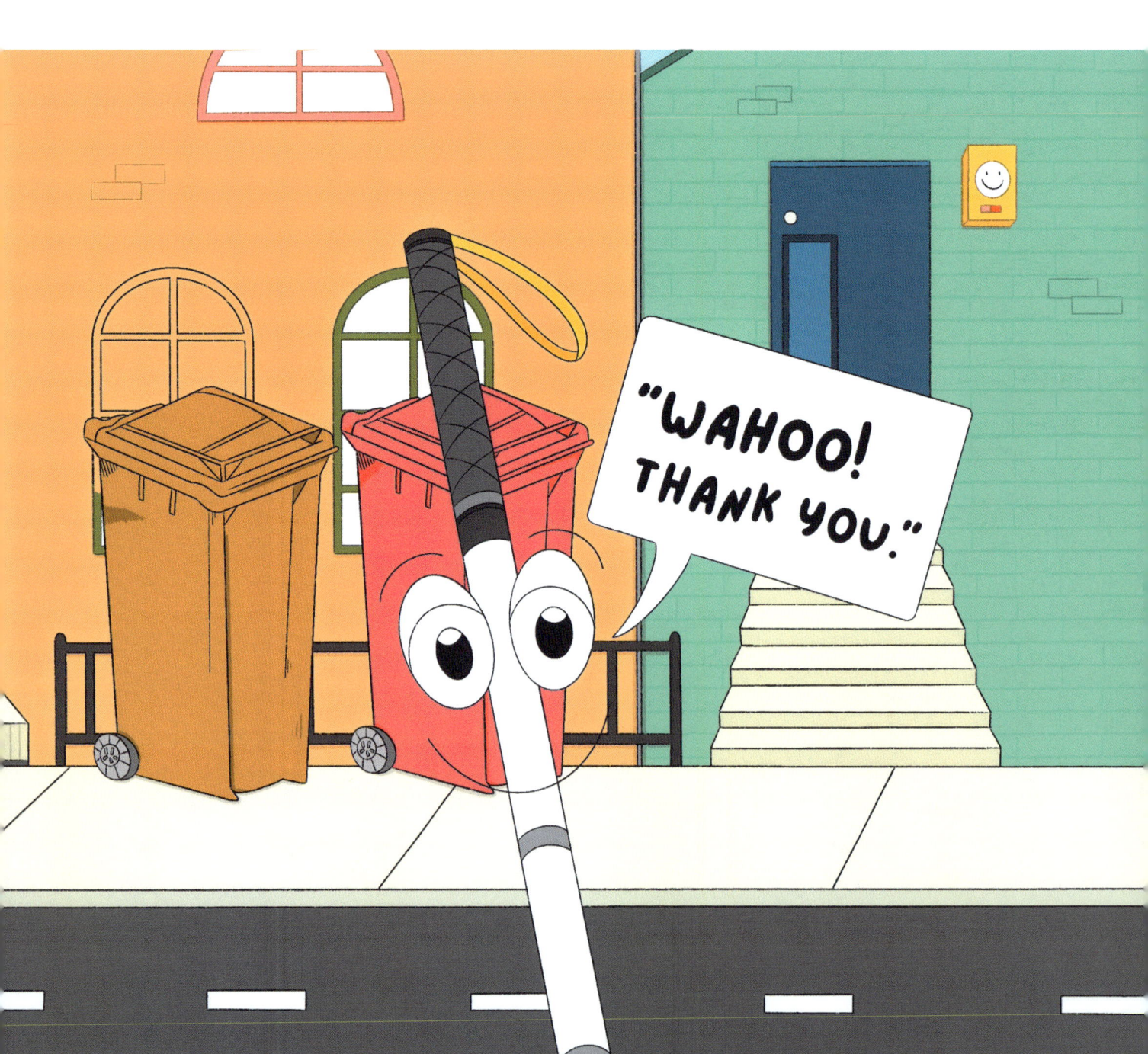

Now that the street is a **BETTER PLACE**, Candy was less battered, bruised and much less smelly.

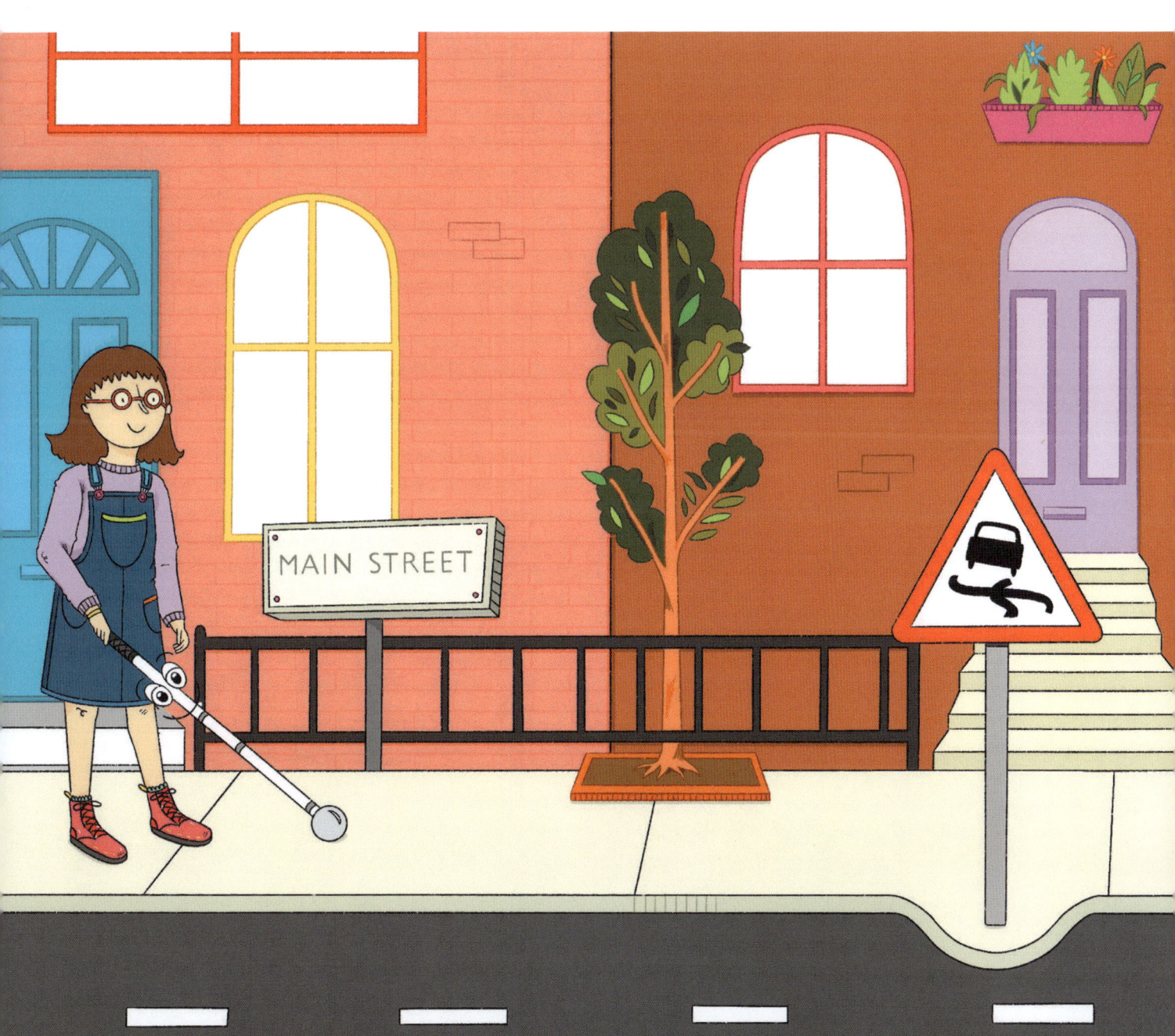

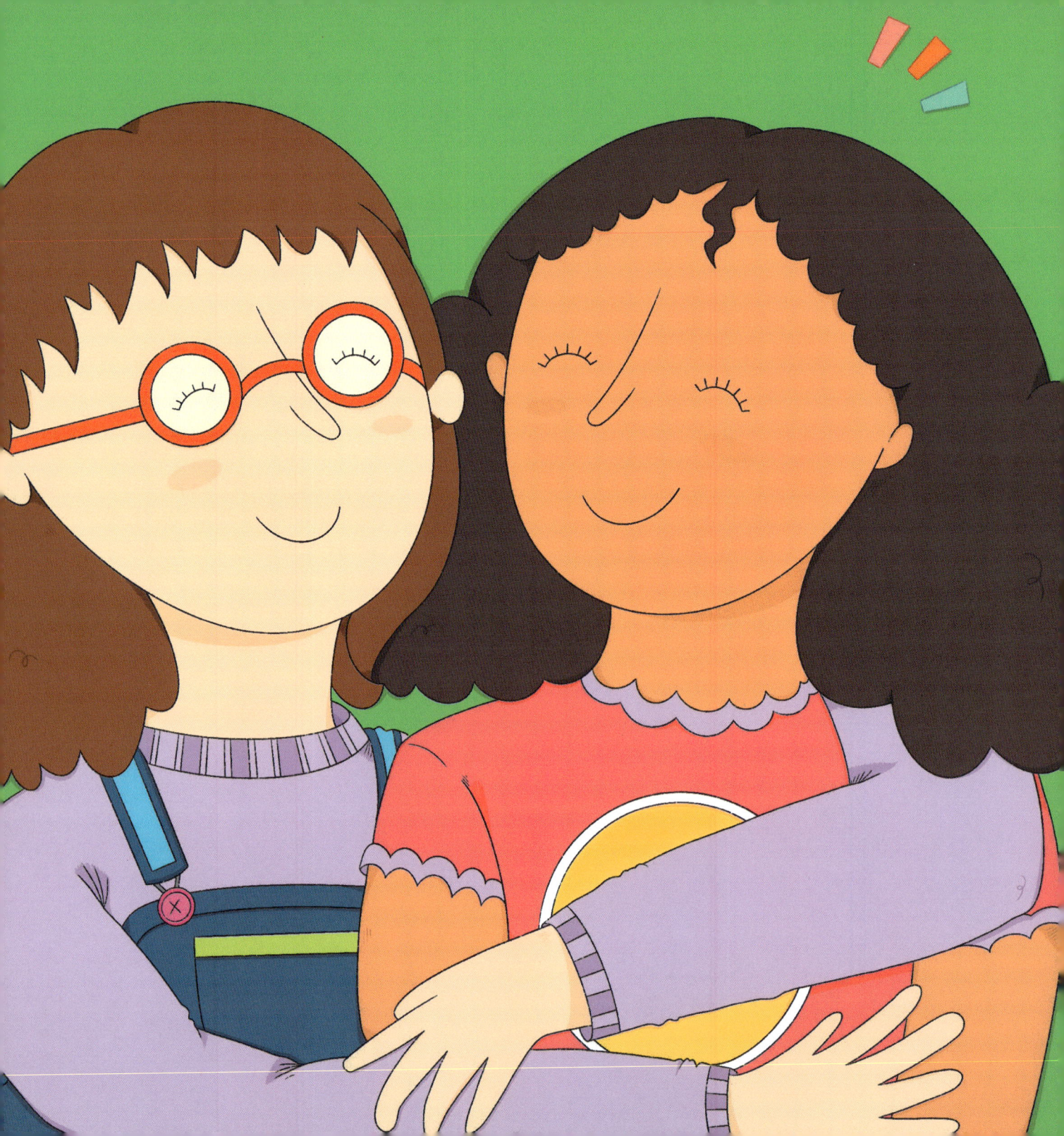

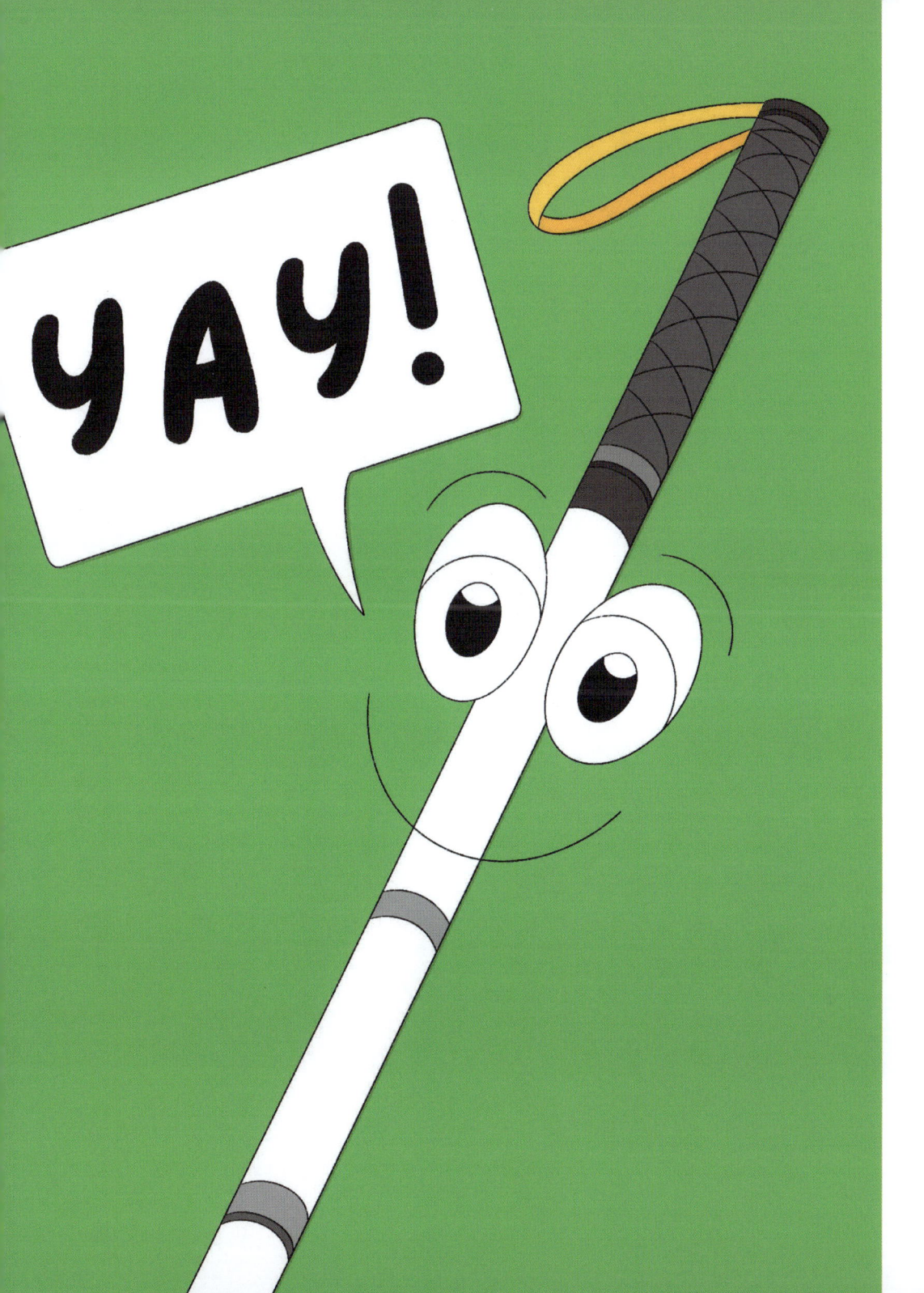

And with a better street, Nicky got to see Kim much more often.

You did great!

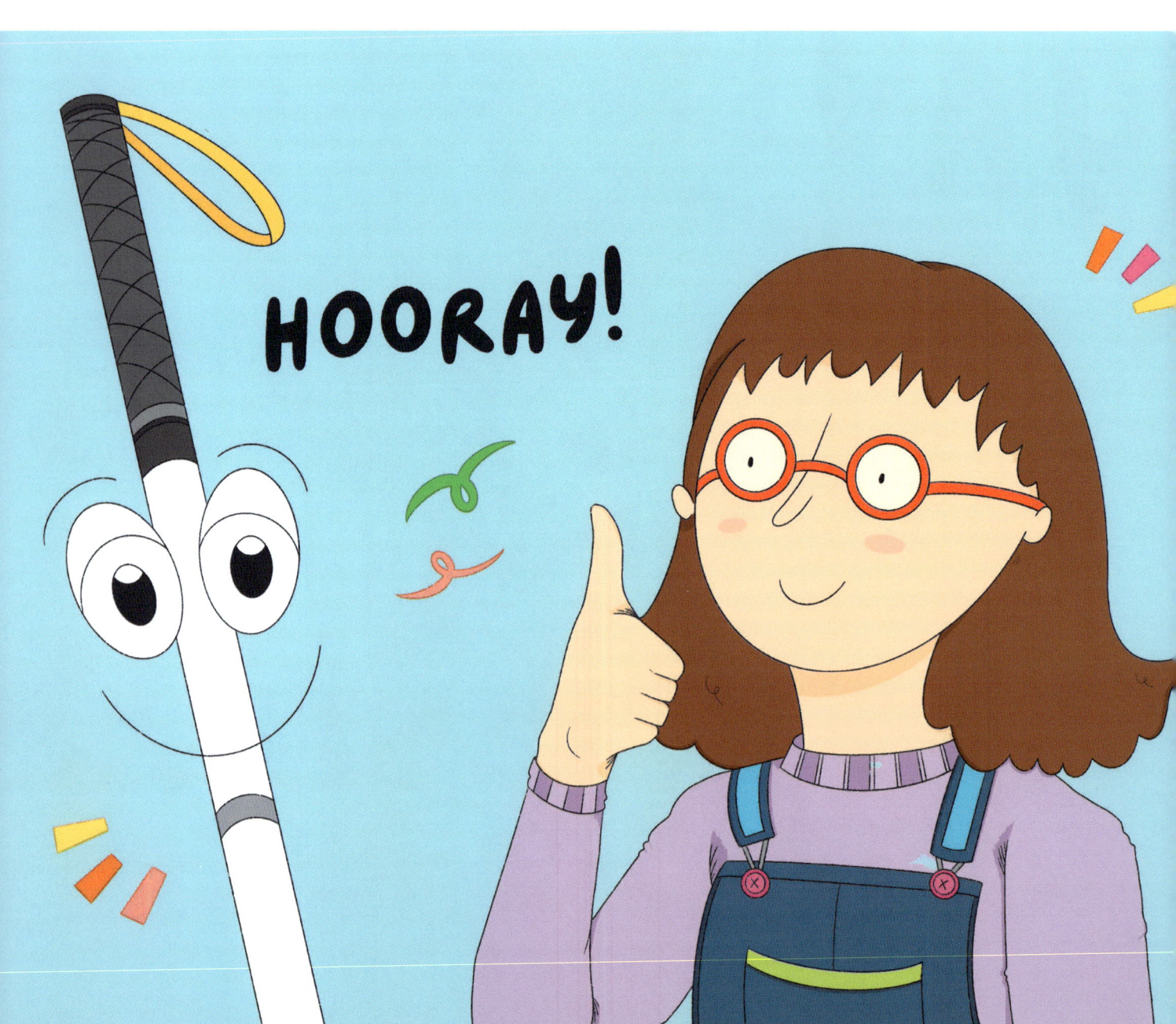

Next time bring your gloves and a bag if you're cleaning up the streets, and make sure you wash your hands afterwards.

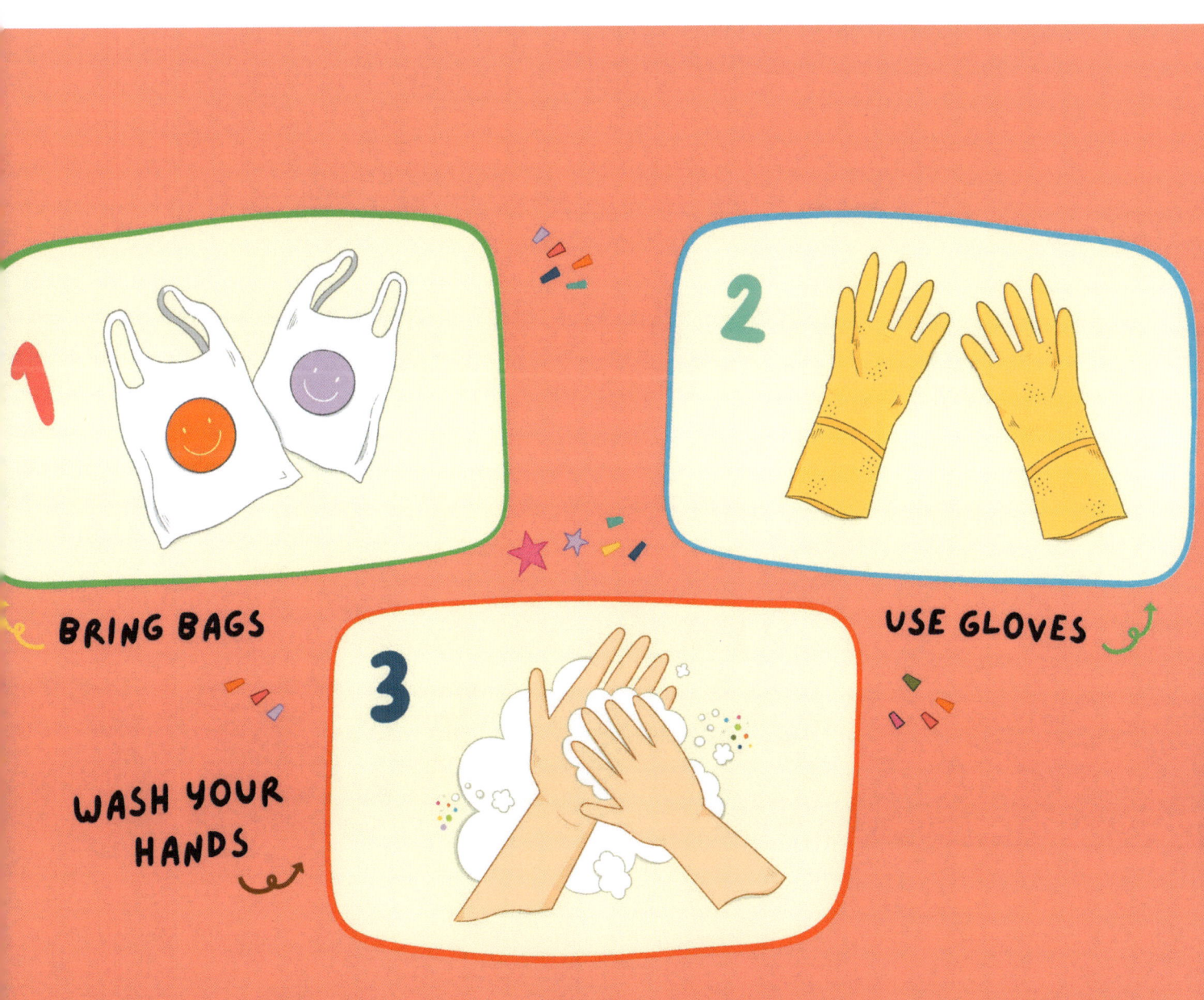

Why not make more places better
by visiting us at

www.betterplaces.uk

where you can find our other books,
activities and resources to help you make

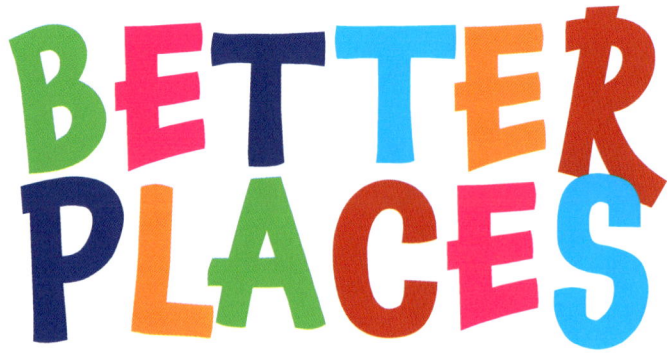

Printed in Great Britain
by Amazon